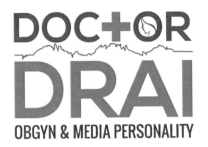

DOC+OR
DRAI
OBGYN & MEDIA PERSONALITY

# 20
## THINGS YOU MAY NOT KNOW ABOUT THE
# PENIS

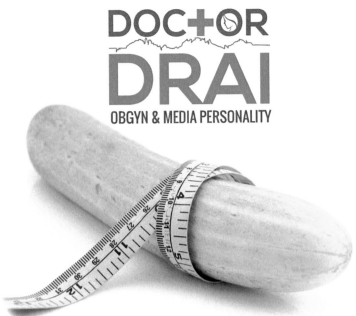

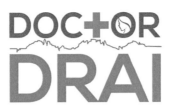

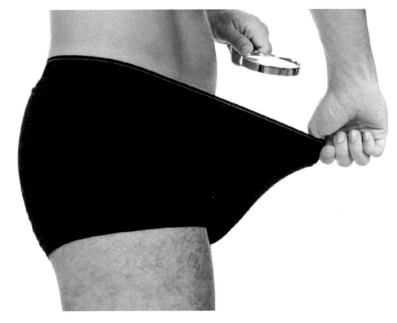

## DEDICATION

### To ALL my #GYNEGirls, #Preggos, and #GENTs:

This book is for YOU, boo. Let me start off by defining #GYNEGirls, #Preggos and #GENTs. You should already know the definitions because you follow me on social media @DrDraiOBGYN and you visit DrDrai.com daily, RIGHT?

Regardless, a #GYNEGirl is a lady who is not pregnant, a #Preggo is a woman who is, and a #GENT is the man that we all LOVE. You ladies ask me questions about your #GENTs' MANHOOD ALL THE TIME. Dr. Drai had no clue there were SOOO many myths out there about the PENIS. So many of ya'll come see me in the office AND haven't the slightest idea of the BASICS about your man's penis.

Listen up! If you don't know your way around DOWN THERE, how are you going to keep your man happy?

Crickets...Crickets...

Because what YOU won't do, another #GYNEGirl (OR #GENT chile) will! After reading this book, you will look at his penis DIFFERENTLY and hopefully know how to WERK it. YASSS! I guess there are some perks for picking a #GayGynecologist as your OBGYN right? LOL!

#GENTS, Dr. Drai didn't leave you HANGING (no pun intended). YOU will learn HOW to use your "tail" to please your lady friend or man friend (no shade) BETTER. TRUST you WILL thank me LATER, Fellas! BTW, penis means, "tail" in Latin in case you were wondering.

To you all, please urge your friends to purchase a copy of this book. A portion of the proceeds will go to one of my favorite charities serving women in domestic violence situations. Domestic violence is REAL. Sadly, I have yet to meet a patient who has not been a victim.

A woman is beaten every 9 seconds in the US. This truly breaks my heart. Remember **if you are in immediate danger, please call 9-1-1.** You can also search **www.domesticshelters.org** to find domestic violence programs in your area OR call the National Domestic Violence Hotline at **1-800-799-7233 (SAFE).** Please pass this info along; you ALREADY know who needs it. Thank you for supporting this important cause.

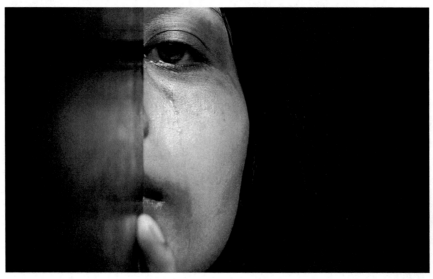

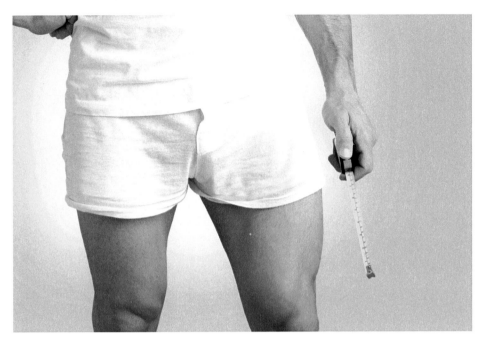

Please enjoy the read. AND Let me know what you think about this #DrDraiMedicalT. In case you didn't know, "Medical T" means Medical TIPs. As a gift to you, for being such great #GYNEGirls, #Preggos & #Gents I created a companion to this book called, '20 Things You May Not Know About the Vagina' and it's free! Go to **DrDrai.com/Vagina** and download your copy today. KISSES...

# TABLE OF CONTENTS

# 20 THINGS YOU MAY NOT KNOW ABOUT THE PENIS

By: Dr. Draion M. Burch, DO
Founder and Chief Medical
Advisor of DrDrai.com

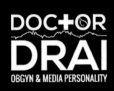

# INTRODUCTION

## For Beginner #GYNEGirls

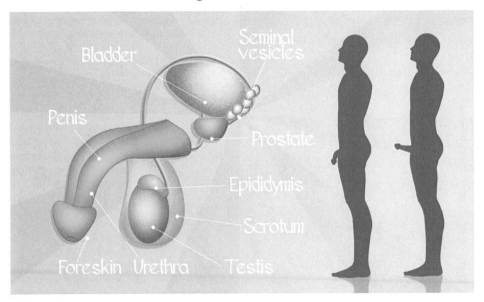

#GYNEGirls, #Preggos, and #GENTs, let's start with the basics.

     HIS PENIS HAS 4 MAIN PARTS:
- Glans (THE HEAD)
- Corpus Cavernosum & Corpus Spongiosum (THE SHAFT)
- The urethra (THE PEE HOLE)

The head is covered by mucosa (AKA a Mucous Lining) that's protected by the foreskin (THE TURTLENECK). If your DOC cuts off the foreskin during a circumcision, the mucosa becomes very dry skin. This is why #GENTs who are uncircumcised has more of a pinkish colored head compared to those who are. The corpus cavernosum is along the side of the penis; when aroused it fills up with blood causing the penis to get HARD.

     BTW the penis is just a BIG ole' clitoris. They are both made of the same tissue. When you suck a penis, it gets hard. If you suck a clitoris, it gets hard too – WINK! However the penis just isn't as sensitive as the clitoris.

It only has 4000 nerves while the clit has 8000. #GirlPower

Now, the corpus spongiosum runs through the center of the penis; the urethra is located in this space. It fills up with blood as well but, not as much as the corpus cavernosum. This is because it has to keep the urethra open. The urethra extends from the bladder. Either semen OR urine can be expelled from it depending upon the situation.

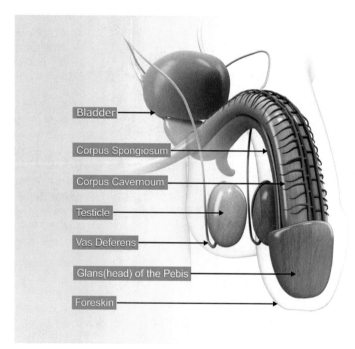

*PENIS ANATOMY*

# For Intermediate #GYNEGirls

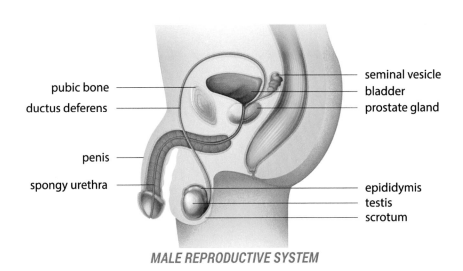

pubic bone
ductus deferens

penis
spongy urethra

seminal vesicle
bladder
prostate gland

epididymis
testis
scrotum

*MALE REPRODUCTIVE SYSTEM*

Let's chat about his other man parts. The scrotum (THE NUT SACK) holds the testes (THE BALLS), which have coiled tubes in them called seminiferous tubules. This is where sperm is made. The male hormone, testosterone, is also made in the testes. On the backside of each of the testes is a tube that stores and matures the sperm called the epididymis.

There is another tube called the vas deferens. It goes from the epididymis, to behind the bladder to connect with the seminal vesicles. This powerful tube helps carry the mature sperm to its final destination- the urethra.

The vas deferens is also the tube that is CUT when your man has a vasectomy. Since we are on this subject, just thought I'd add, it's always easier for a man to get his tubes cut than a woman. BUT, Dr. Drai will save that rant for another book.

The seminal vesicles are grape-like structures that are attached to the vas deferens near the bladder. It secretes the fluid that makes up most of the semen. This fluid contains fructose, the sugar that gives sperm energy so they can move. It also has alkaline properties that protects the sperm and prolongs their life when they are deposited inside the acidic environment of the vagina. The place where the vas deferens and seminal vesicles meet is called the ejaculatory duct.

# For Advanced #GYNEGirls

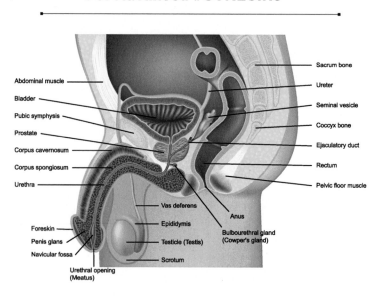

Sacrum bone

Abdominal muscle

Ureter

Bladder

Seminal vesicle

Pubic symphysis

Coccyx bone

Prostate

Ejaculatory duct

Corpus cavernosum

Corpus spongiosum

Rectum

Urethra

Pelvic floor muscle

Vas deferens

Anus

Epididymis

Foreskin

Bulbourethral gland (Cowper's gland)

Penis glans

Testicle (Testis)

Navicular fossa

Scrotum

Urethral opening (Meatus)

*MALE REPRODUCTIVE SYSTEM*

The ejaculatory duct carries the NOW semen to the urethra. It also meets the urethra in the prostate gland.

The prostate gland is a walnut sized structure that produces fluid to help nourish the sperm. This fluid has enzymes, zinc, and citric acid in it. The most important enzyme in this fluid is Prostate Specific Antigen (PSA); it liquefies semen to allow the sperm to swim freely.

Additionally, there is another gland called the Bulbourethral gland (Cowper's gland) that also makes fluid for the sperm. It empties directly into the urethra. The fluid made here is alkaline and contains mucous. This fluid is also called pre-ejaculate, you know Pre-Cum. Pre-Cum neutralizes the acid in urine. It also lubricates the urethra protecting the sperm from being damaged.

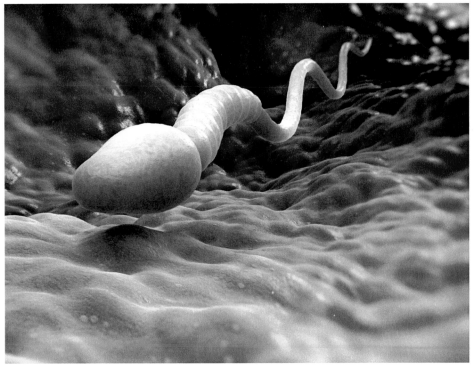

*SPERM*

Now that we know all of his parts- let's discuss how sperm travels a little more in depth. Sperm is made in the testes and stored and matured in the epididymis. The sperm then travels through the vas deferens to the ejaculatory duct. It then travels from the ejaculatory duct to the urethra. During this process, the seminal vesicles, prostate gland, and Cowper's gland all add extra fluid to sperm to nourish them.

### SPERM + Extra Fluid = SEMEN! Get it?

Have you ever wondered why men don't pee and ejaculate (nut) at the same time? During ejaculation, there's a sphincter at the base of the bladder that squeezes the urethra to close it. So, there's no urine in semen AND no semen in the bladder. Isn't the male anatomy amazing? BTW, the farthest recorded distance a man has ever ejaculated was 18 feet. WOW!

# PENILE CANCER

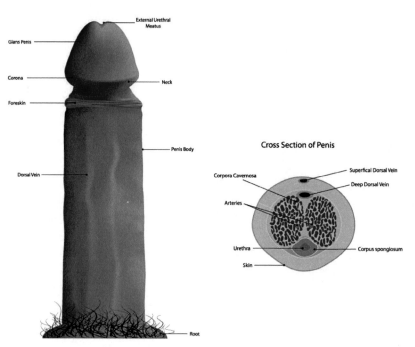

Penile cancer is very rare; it occurs in less than 1 in 100,000 #Gents and accounts for less than 1% of cancers in men in the US. The average age of a man when diagnosed is 68. Penile cancer can appear anywhere on the penis however it usually occurs in the foreskin or the head. In the US, it is estimated that this year 1800 men will be diagnosed with penile cancer and about 300 will die. Men with Human Papilloma Virus (HPV), those who are uncircumcised, and smokers, have a higher risk for developing this type of cancer.

Men should ALWAYS wear a condom to protect themselves against HPV and other sexually transmitted infections (STIs). #GENTs, if your naked penis touches a cervix that has HPV on it, you will get that virus on the head of

---

*Side note: Just stop smoking; I know it's tough. Dr. Drai quit "cold turkey" because he had his mind made up. You have to figure out why you smoke. I smoked when stressed out. So instead of picking up a cigarette, I went to the GYM AND I saved LOTs of money. Plus I'm super FINE. LOL! Ya'll know it's expensive to smoke. Find out why you smoke and then substitute that why with something healthy. Sorry I got sidetracked...*

your penis. #GYNEGirls, that goes for you too; if a man has HPV on the head of his penis and it touches your cervix during sex, you will get HPV on your cervix. #WrapItUp! #TeamCondoms! Where do you think cervical cancer comes from? #BoysBoysBoys! Don't forget #GYNEGirls AND #Gents; you need to get that HPV vaccine; this gives you added protection against cervical cancer AND penile cancer.

#GENTs-if you see or feel anything weird on your shaft, talk to your doctor. Let me be more specific—if you see sores, blisters, warts, lumps, skin thickening or ulcers, please make an appointment ASAP. These are all symptoms of Penile Cancer. The most common symptom is changes in the skin on your penis. Your doctor will need to take a biopsy to make a proper diagnosis. If caught early, the 5 year survival rate is super HIGH- 85%. If your doctor thinks the cancer has spread to other body parts, you will need a biopsy of your lymph nodes and imaging done of your entire body. Treatment options include surgery, chemotherapy, and/or radiation depending on how advanced the cancer is, your health, and your personal preferences. PLEASE communicate with your DOC #GENTs!

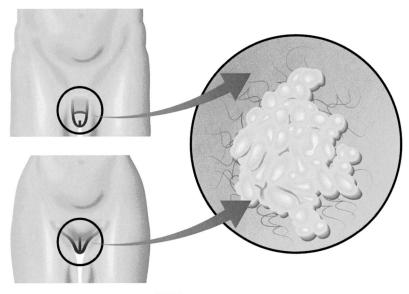

*HPV*
*HUMAN PAILLOMAVIRUS*

# TESTICULAR CANCER

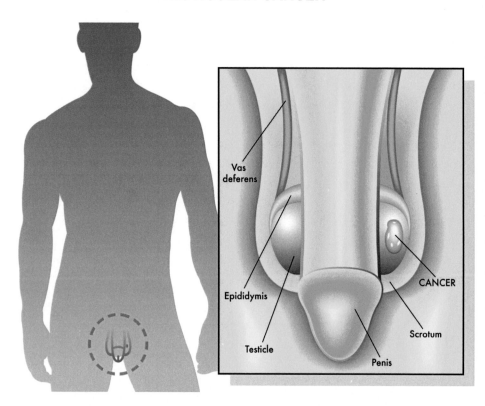

Testicular cancer is the most common cancer affecting males between the ages of 15-35. It accounts for only 1% of all cancers in men. In the US, it's estimated that this year 8000 men will be diagnosed with testicular cancer and about 300 will die. #Gents with an un-descended testicle, those having a family history of testicular cancer, men that are tall, Caucasian, or have had cancer in 1 testicle are at risk.

Testicular cancer is one of the most curable cancers. #GYNEGirls, your man may complain of a lump, painless swelling in 1 testicle, aching in the belly, around the anus, or scrotum. Some men will have sudden pain in the groin or gynecomastia (man boobs). If your #BAE has any of these symptoms, take off of work and take him to your primary care physician, immediately. Your DOC will order some blood tests and an ultrasound to look for signs of cancer.

If concerned about the cancer spreading throughout your body, your DOC will order other imaging studies. He actually will have to have surgery to diagnose this; the testicle of concern is removed. This surgery can also treat the cancer though. That's a plus. If cancer is found treatment options include surgery, chemotherapy, and/or radiation. Luckily, the cure rate is HIGH.

There are actually no medical studies that support you checking the testes for possible cancer, therefore many medical organizations DO NOT recommend checking "the boys" regularly unless he is experiencing pain. That's why Dr. Drai wants you to know your man's parts. Make sure you #GYNEGirls, "check" your man's balls. Feel for lumps, hardness, or swelling. #GENTs, you can check deez nuts too – WINK!

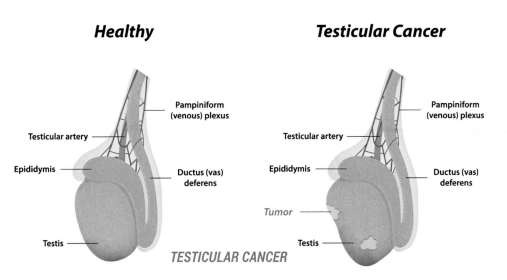

**Healthy**

**Testicular Cancer**

Pampiniform (venous) plexus

Testicular artery

Epididymis

Ductus (vas) deferens

Testis

TESTICULAR CANCER

Pampiniform (venous) plexus

Testicular artery

Epididymis

Ductus (vas) deferens

Tumor

Testis

## OTHER BALL BUSTERS...

#GYNEGirls, let's chat about other ball busters. This is a common scenario: your man goes to the doctor and was given a diagnosis of varicocele. Then you come into MY office and ask me 50 million questions about it; after you have already checked with Dr. Google first... (shaking my head). Stop believing everything you read online. LOL! With that said, let's ALL get on the same page.

## VARICOCELE

A varicocele is a group of dilated veins in the scrotum. This can cause your #GENT to have issues with his sperm. Oddly, your man won't have any symptoms and this usually only becomes an issue when you are trying to become #Preggo. This is why it is important for your man to also be examined AND "worked-up" for infertility problems too. It's not always you, ladies. Surgery is needed ONLY if pain, infertility, or testicular atrophy (shrinking of balls) occurs.

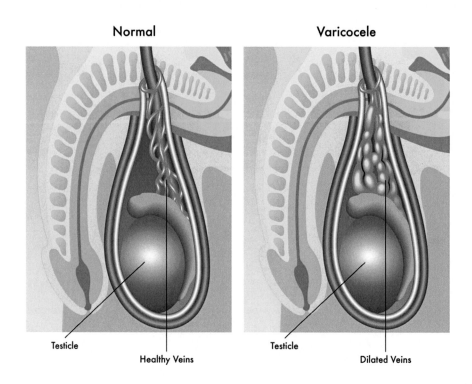

Normal      Varicocele

Testicle     Testicle

Healthy Veins     Dilated Veins

# HYDROCELE

**Healthy Testicle**

Pampiniform
(venous) plexus

Testicular artery

Epididymis

Ductus (vas)
deferens

Testis

**Hydrocele**

Pampiniform
(venous) plexus

Testicular artery

Epididymis

Accumulation
of fluid

Ductus (vas)
deferens

Testis

A hydrocele is a fluid-filled sac surrounding a testicle causing some swelling in the scrotum. Your man will complain of painless swelling in his sack. In adults, this can be caused from inflammation or infection "down there." Hydroceles usually do not affect fertility. Surgery is needed ONLY if it's large enough to cause pain.

# EPIDIDYMITIS

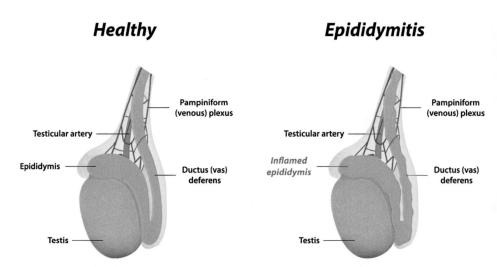

Epididymitis is an inflammation of the epididymis that is usually caused by a STI like chlamydia or gonorrhea. Your #BAE may complain of swollen nuts, pain in the testicles or lower abdomen, pain with urination or ejaculation, discharge from the penis or even blood in the semen. Antibiotics, ice packs, jock straps, and ibuprofen should relieve some of the inflammation! STIs...Please ain't nobody got time for THAT!

## PROSTATE CANCER

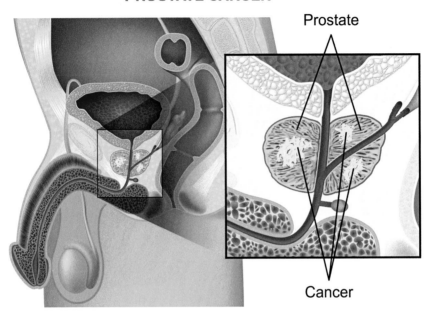

Prostate

Cancer

Prostate cancer is the second most common cancer found in American men. In the US, it's estimated that this year 220,000 men will be diagnosed with Prostate cancer and about 27,000 will die. #GYNEGirls, your #GENT may have problems with urination or blood in his urine or semen. These problems are usually associated with men who have non-cancerous enlargement of their prostate (officially known as Benign Prostatic Hyperplasia aka BPH), however it's hard to tell the difference between this AND cancer.

If your man has any of these symptoms, take him to your primary care doctor ASAP. Being obese, African-American, older, eating lots of red meat and dairy products, and having a family history of breast or prostate cancer puts your man at a higher risk for getting prostate cancer. Get healthy fellas- eat more fruits and veggies AND exercise daily. Digital rectal exams (DRE) should be done annually to examine the prostate for men over age 50.

Bend over Boys!

Just teasing...

## PROSTATE EXAM

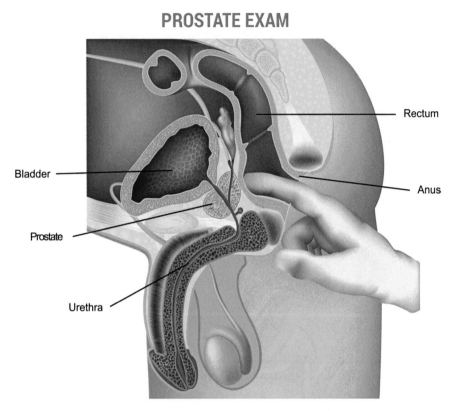

African American men or men who have had a father, brother, or son with prostate cancer are advised to get their prostate checked a bit earlier, at age 45. Your doctor may order a prostate-specific antigen (PSA) test. It's nothing more than a simple blood test fellas. PSA is a substance that is naturally produced by the prostate gland. It becomes elevated when the prostate is irritated by inflammation or infection, becomes enlarged, or has cancer.

If your DOC is concerned about prostate cancer based on your exam and blood tests, you will get an ultrasound of the prostate done and a biopsy. If cancer has spread to other body parts, you will need a biopsy of your lymph nodes and imaging done of your entire body. Treatment options include observation, cryotherapy, vaccine treatment, hormone therapy, surgery, chemotherapy, and/or radiation depending on the how advanced the cancer is, your health, and your personal preferences.

# OTHER PROSTATE PROBLEMS...

**Normal Prostate**

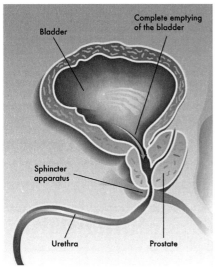

**Prostatic Hypertrophy**

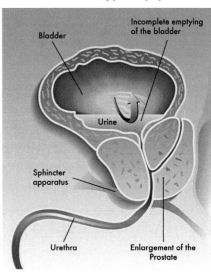

*BENIGN PROSTATIC HYPERPLASIA (BPH)*

The symptoms of BPH are the same as prostate cancer. Diabetes and heart disease with the use of beta blockers (drugs used to lower blood pressure) increases your risk of having BPH. Treatment depends upon the size of the prostate, your age, your overall health, and whether or not the enlarged prostate is problematic. Medications such as Flomax (Tamsulosin), Cardura (Doxazosin), Proscar (Finasteride), and Cialis (Tadalafil) may help. If not, surgery is the next option.

# PROSTATITIS

Prostatitis is an infection or inflammation in the prostate gland. If bacteria suddenly infects the prostate, your #GENT may complain of a bladder infection, urinating a lot (especially at night), fever, chills, nausea, or vomiting. He may also have pelvic pain. To treat these symptoms he will need antibiotics, pain meds, and lots of fluids.

Chronic prostatitis can occur after having many bladder infections. BTW, most prostatitis is chronic, meaning lasting more than 3 months and is not caused by a bacterial infection. Men usually complain of genital or bladder pain. The symptoms are not as bad as the ones mentioned above, however, he may need to take antibiotics for a longer time (up to 12 weeks).

## Normal prostate

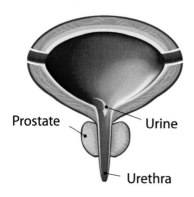

Prostate — Urine

— Urethra

## Prostatitis

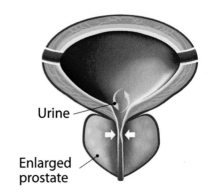

Urine —

Enlarged prostate

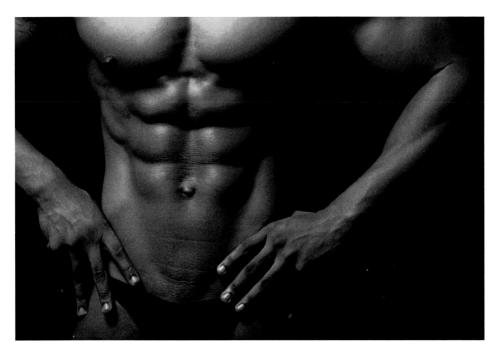

Now that I've gained your attention with the basics—I hope you've learned a lot from the introduction. Chocolate...YUMMY. I'm in LOVE with the #COCO. LOL!

## Medical T (TIPs) #1 - The Putrid Penis

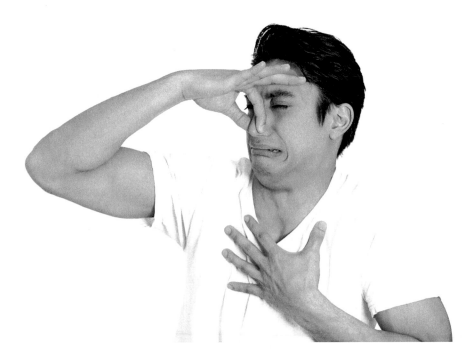

Sweaty balls, moisture, and natural bacteria means ODOR, chile! A putrid odor...Puuuu-weee! Some of ya'll find the smell of your man's genitals arousing though, #Pheromones. If that's not the case, teach him how to "manscape."

Too much pubic hair can keep it DAMP down there. Hunni, DAMP means bacteria. Those little buggers love to grow in moist places. Trim his pubes with clippers – the ones with adjustable guards. However, don't let him shave until he's BARE. Your man might get those annoying ingrown hairs, which can lead to infection and scarring.

Wash his privates with a gentle antibacterial soap. If your #BAE is uncircumcised (ya know has a turtleneck) pull the foreskin back to clean the head properly. Get under those balls, boo! AND don't forget about his anus. It needs to be washed too – with a different washcloth of course.

To dry his genitals off, try a blow dryer. If the entire area is not dry, he will trap moisture and this putrid cycle begins, AGAIN. Make sure he is changing his bath towels on a regular basis. Towels can be full of bacteria. Hunni, if your man has that smell REAL BAD, put some deodorant under those balls.

That's Dr. Drai's FAVORITE "Medical T." Skip the deodorant though, if you are planning to give him some oral action.

Additionally, trade his silk jock strap (LOL!) in for cotton boxers. Cotton is best to block out moisture. He also needs to wash his gym clothes. These #GENTs wear those same workout clothes for weeks. Don't forget to air out those gym shoes too.

#GYNEGirls, your man may be a lil' apprehensive about these changes, but have fun with it. Create a day spa for him. #GENTs LOVE to be pampered too ladies!

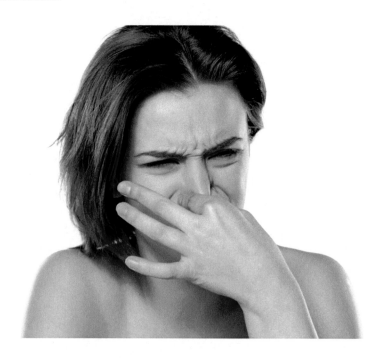

# MEDICAL NOTES

_____

_____

_____

_____

_____

_____

_____

_____

_____

_____

_____

_____

_____

# MEDICAL NOTES

_____

_____

_____

_____

_____

_____

_____

_____

_____

_____

_____

_____

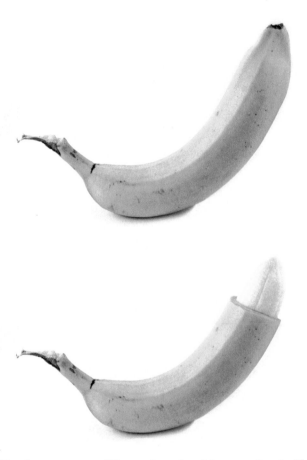

#GYNEGIRLs, let me start off by saying that it's completely NATURAL for a #GENT to have his banana suit, aka foreskin. The foreskin, also known as the prepuce, is a loose fold of skin that covers and protects the head of the penis AND the urethral meatus (pee hole opening) when it's soft. It's similar to the clitoral hood; the skin that covers your clit.

No worries! It's retractable ladies. You can move it back and forth but do it gently, please. This skin is very delicate and can tear easily. There is however, a medical condition called phimosis where the foreskin won't retract. It usually resolves over time but can cause balanitis; an infection of the foreskin. Another medical condition called paraphimosis can also occur where the foreskin gets swollen and trapped behind the head when it is pulled back. This can cut off the blood flow to the head of the penis, which can lead to gangrene. Chile this one is NO JOKE! This is a medical emergency that requires immediate surgery.

Ok, enough about foreskin retraction drama. Sometimes when the penis is erect, you can't even tell that your man has foreskin. The cool thing about this magical tissue is that it's covered with an inner moist mucous membrane that provides natural lubrication for the tip of his penis. It is also used to grow eyelids for burn victims. Interesting right?

Have you even seen an uncircumcised ADULT penis soft? Well y'all act like you haven't! The truth is that most men in the world ARE NOT circumcised, ladies! Circumcision is an American thing.

You #Preggos always say that you want your baby circumcised so he won't get teased in the locker room during his teen years. Dr. Drai gets it! So let's chat about circumcision.

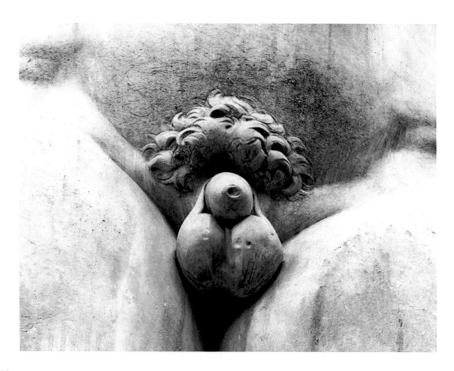

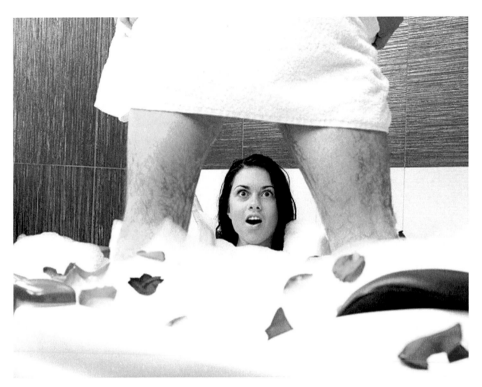

Circumcision is the surgical removal of the foreskin. This is done for religious, but mostly cosmetic reasons. Actually circumcision was originally thought to prevent men from masturbating...yeah that really worked right? LOL!

As soon as you find out you are having a BOY at your 18-20 week anatomy ultrasound (or even earlier these days), you need to sit down with your OBGYN, Family Medicine DOC, or Midwife to discuss circumcision. Babies born with bleeding problems, anomalies with their penis, or are considered medically unstable CANNOT be circumcised. What are anomalies in the penis, you ask? Let me explain.

Hypospadias is a birth defect where the urethral opening (pee pee hole) is not located in the center of the glans. Chordee is another defect. This is when the head of the penis curves downward. Both have to be corrected surgically by an urologist AND circumcision must be avoided in BOTH cases.

Circumcision has its benefits. It lowers rates of Urinary Tract Infections (UTIs), penile cancer, STIs and makes it easier to clean the penis. AND there are none of those retraction issues. But, there are RISKS involved with circumcision: bleeding, infection, damage to the head of the penis or the urethra opening, and cutting too much foreskin off.

To bring this "Medical T" to a head (no pun intended), let me clear one thing up: There is no difference in sexual satisfaction between men who have been circumcised versus men who have not. You ladies always ask me

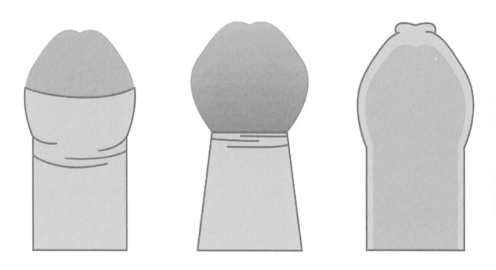

about this. And another thing...Hand jobs are WAY different for the #GENT with foreskin. Because of that extra skin, there's more of a gliding motion and less friction with stroking. You still need to use lube though. Here's my FAVORITE "Medical T."

Use your tongue to tickle the inside of his foreskin; it's very sensitive. Thank me later. Now, enough with ALL of these foreskin follies. Next chapter! And of course, Dr. Drai left you with some more EYE candy!

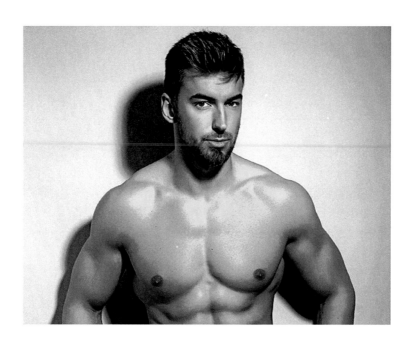

# MEDICAL NOTES

_____

_____

_____

_____

_____

_____

_____

_____

_____

_____

_____

_____

# MEDICAL NOTES

_____

_____

_____

_____

_____

_____

_____

_____

_____

_____

_____

_____

_____

_____

# Medical T (TIPs) #3 - The Curved Cock

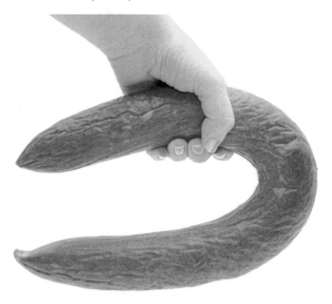

I know y'all are cracking up with this title. BUT it's no laughing matter. #GYNEGirls and #GENTs, let's keep it real. You have all seen a curved cock before right? A slight curve can be normal. But there are instances where the curve is as severe as the sausage above.

Have you ever heard a #GENT say that his _ick will curve to your vagina? There's some truth in that! It's called Peyronie's disease (PD).

PD is when there is scar tissue along the side of the penis that causes painful curved hard-ons. You can actually feel the scar on their penis. It feels like a lump or something hard. #GENTs who suffer from PD have trouble maintaining an erection. Sex is painful and their cock can shorten during an erection due to this.

We don't know EXACTLY why this happens but, it is thought to be caused by repeated injuries. There's damage to the penis and a scar forms during the healing process. When your BOO is aroused, the area where the scar is won't stretch so the penis bends. OUCH! And don't bring him to me HUNNI! Go to an urologist ASAP!

Depending on how bad it is, they may observe his condition, try medications, or go to surgery. #GYNEGirls, be compassionate if this is happening to your #BAE. Promise me? Here's one of my FAVORITE "Medical T's" for you. If his penis is curved downwards (toward the ground), ride him backwards- reverse cowgirl (or cowboy no shade) to get yours. The tip of the penis will touch your "G-spot" goodies. All curved cocks aren't created equal.

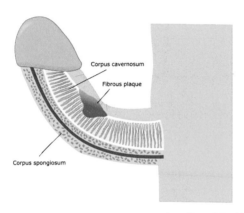 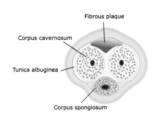

**PEYONE'S DISEASE**

# MEDICAL ☕ NOTES

_____

_____

_____

_____

_____

_____

_____

_____

_____

_____

_____

_____

# MEDICAL NOTES

_____

_____

_____

_____

_____

_____

_____

_____

_____

_____

_____

_____

_____

## Medical T (TIPs) #4 - The Average Joe

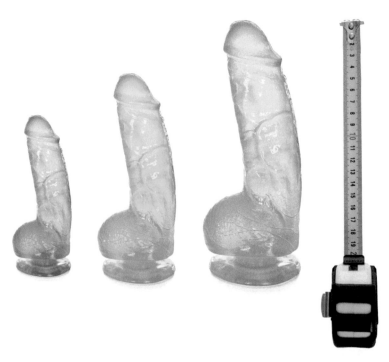

Here is an age-old question: What's the size of the average penis? I ask because #GENTs are obsessed with the size of their penises. It's not about how BIG it is, it's about what you DO with what you've got. Can I get an AMEN, ladies? Right...

Studies say that most women are happy with their man's penis size but #GENTs are not. Why? Well first of all, ALL men watch PORN. Let me say that again... ALL MEN WATCH PORN. This creates a problem because the men that a #GENT is modeling his bedroom behavior after have 10+ inch penises when hard. When have you ever seen a man with a small penis being featured in a porn flick? EXACTLY...

The second issue that causes your #GENT to be anxious about his penis size is the point of view. Men are looking down at their penis so it will seem small. Women are looking at their man's penis face on. Plus it's erect. So of course it looks HUGE. Sometimes having longer pubes can make it seem even smaller if looking from the top down.

Third, men have bigger hands than women. When they are jerking their turkey, their hands completely surround their penis...sometimes. This can add to their thought that Mr. Big is actually Mr. Small. The #GENTs with the big ones have to use two hands — WINK!

By the way, you never can tell how long his thang is going to get when it's aroused. Don't assume #GYNEGirls. The average length of the penis ranges from 2.8-3.9 inches when SOFT and 4.7-6.3 inches when HARD. The average girth of the penis is 3.5-3.9 inches when SOFT and about 4.7 inches when HARD.

Here's another one of Dr. Drai's FAVORITE "Medical T's." When you are riding on top of an average Joe, GRIND chile. Stop all of that jumping up and down business. When you grind, his penis head is constantly hitting the right spot. It's okay to be an average JOE, fellas... When the #GENTs come in with their wives, baby mamas, fiancés, or girlfriends, I always tell them

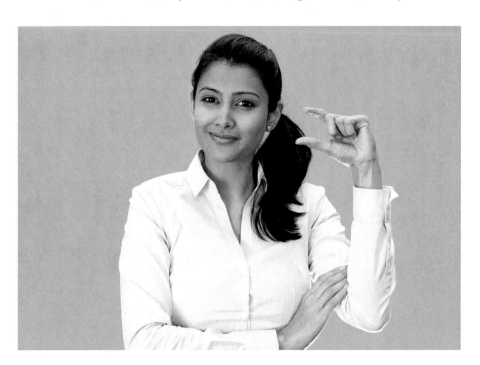

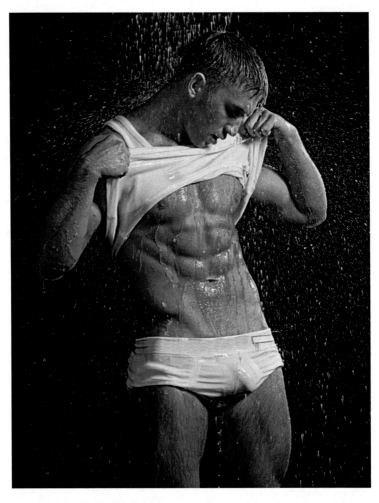

about this one study. Men worry about the length BUT women worry about the GIRTH. So, #GENTs, if your manhood is as FAT as a mug, you are good!

# MEDICAL ☕ NOTES

_____

_____

_____

_____

_____

_____

_____

_____

_____

_____

_____

_____

_____

# MEDICAL NOTES

_____

_____

_____

_____

_____

_____

_____

_____

_____

_____

_____

_____

# Medical T (TIPs) #5 - One (Nut) is Enough!

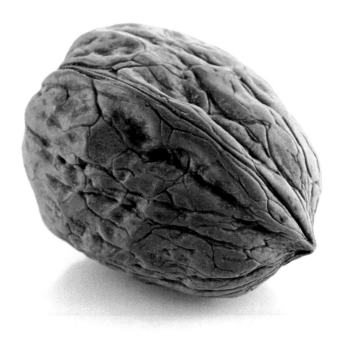

Lots of you come see me in the office and ask, "Can I get pregnant if my man only has 1 ball?" The answer is YES, ladies. #GENTs with monorchism (one nut wonders) have more than enough testosterone to make sperm. There are several situations that can cause your boo to be 1-sided.

When male babies are in the belly, their testes descend into the scrotum. Sometimes, as I mentioned in the introduction, 1 ball doesn't travel that far. When birthed, the baby only has 1 testicle. This is called cryptorchidism. We can usually feel the un-descended ball in the groin. You definitely want that nut removed because there is a risk of testicular cancer if left behind.

Fellas that play rough sports can also lose a ball. No pun intended. The testicle can twist (torsion) and die; so it has to be removed. This is SOOO painful. Some of you #GYNEGirls joke about busting your man's balls, but in this situation leave the only ball he has left alone. PLEASE! He could lose it too if you injure it.

Here's my Favorite "Medical T": During oral sex, don't forget to put his ball(s) completely in your mouth one by one AND lightly suck. Oh and lick that line in the middle of his nut sack; it's called the raphe. That's a hot spot. WINK!

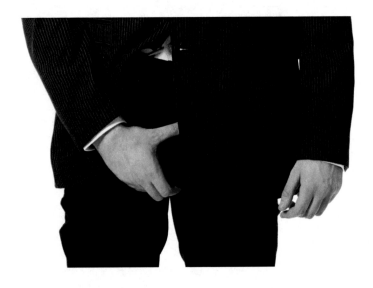

Side note 1
*If someone does hit him in his junk, he will feel it in his stomach because the same nerves bring feelings to both areas.*

Side note 2
*You may not even know that he was missing a ball. We now have testicular implants.*

# MEDICAL ☕ NOTES

_____

_____

_____

_____

_____

_____

_____

_____

_____

_____

_____

_____

_____

_____

# MEDICAL NOTES

_____

_____

_____

_____

_____

_____

_____

_____

_____

_____

_____

_____

_____

# Medical T (TIPs) #6 - The Male G-Spot

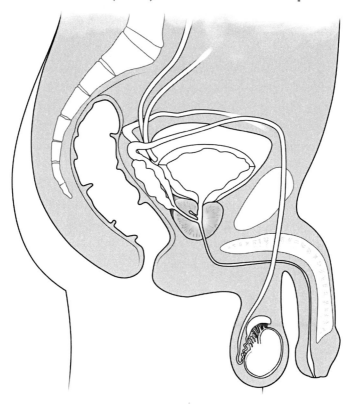

#GYNEGirls, let's chat for a minute. You all complain that you get tired of the same ole' sex routine with your man. Do you want to learn how to spice things up and keep him "cuming" and coming for more? Well let Dr. Drai teach you about the Male G-Spot, aka the PROSTATE GLAND. This "Medical T" is sure to do the trick!

    The Prostate gland is shaped like a walnut and is located 2 inches in his bum. It is not difficult to find. If your man is a bit freaky, you can try to put your fingers in his rectum to locate it. This is risky! You never know how he's going to react. If you dare to be daring and try this, be sure to cut your nails and proceed with caution. You may want to rim him (anilingus, aka eat the booty) to loosen him up. Don't forget the lube!

For the tight ended #Gents, next time you are giving him some oral play I want you to apply upward pressure with your fingers on his taint, the space between his balls and anus. You can put a vibrator in that spot too. This will stimulate his prostate as well.

Ladies, before you indulge in butt play, please make sure it's clean AND you use protection- dental dam and latex gloves. You can get STIs from rimming, BOO BOO. This is the only time I suggest using a douche. Fellas just put some water in the rectum in an old enema bottle. Your lady will appreciate your efforts. And relax, just because you let your #BAE finger your BUTT doesn't make you gay OR a bottom. Couldn't leave my gay #GENTs out...

Another way to stimulate the prostate is to use a butt plug? What is a butt plug you ask? A butt plug is a sex toy designed to go inside the rectum. It puts pressure on the prostate gland to heighten sexual arousal. You can also insert a dildo in the rectum to achieve the same result. However, if you going

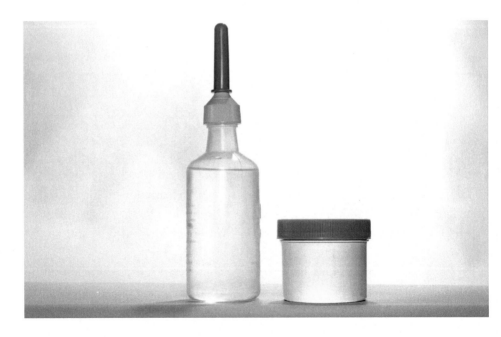

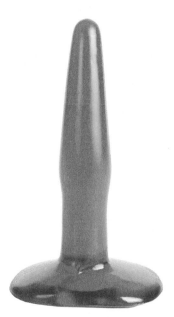

to use a dildo, make sure it's smaller than his penis. There should be only one Mandingo in your bedroom and it's your man.

This is one of my FAVORITE "Medical T." Make sure that any toys you purchase are 100% medical grade silicone. There are no pores in this material so bacteria can't live there and cause infection. Use lube and condoms with your toys, too. Are you ready ladies? Now go find his G-spot!

# MEDICAL NOTES

_____

_____

_____

_____

_____

_____

_____

_____

_____

_____

_____

_____

_____

# MEDICAL NOTES

_____

_____

_____

_____

_____

_____

_____

_____

_____

_____

_____

_____

_____

## Medical T (TIPs) #7 - The Broken Boner

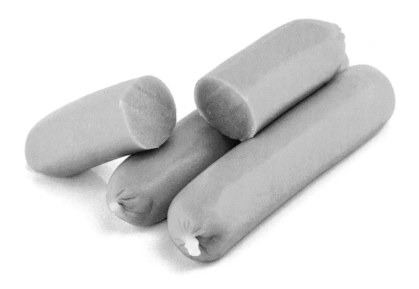

This chapter is PAINFUL. Did you know the penis can break? It sure can, #GYNEGirls. It's called a penis fracture. If the penis is bent forcefully while hard, the lining of the penis will break. You can actually hear it break; it will sound like a POP. When this happens, the penis will have dark bruising because blood is moving out of the capsule. This may cause him to urinate blood and his pee hole may be damaged as well. This is a medical emergency requiring immediate surgery. If he doesn't get treated, his penis may not work again.

This can happen if he aggressively masturbates or is having rough sex. Dr. Drai has seen this situation TWICE too many times. Both times that I have seen this in the ER, the woman was riding his penis – HARD.

Here's my FAVORITE "Medical T." Ladies, you have to ride in the direction that his penis is curved so this won't happen. For example, if his penis is straight, hump up and down. If his penis is curved up, hump from front to back. You get the picture.

Remember ladies, sex doesn't have to be so ROUGH. Say NO to a broken boner... Next chapter!

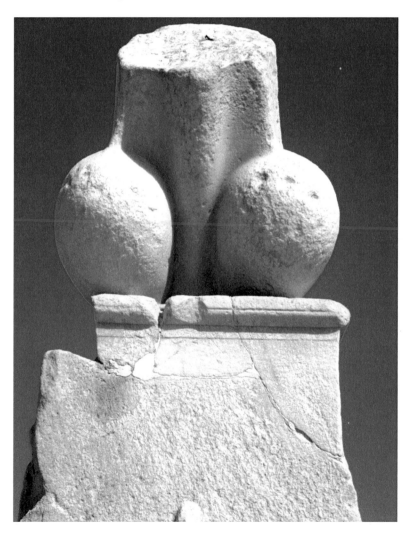

# MEDICAL NOTES

_____

_____

_____

_____

_____

_____

_____

_____

_____

_____

_____

_____

# MEDICAL ☕ NOTES

_____

_____

_____

_____

_____

_____

_____

_____

_____

_____

_____

_____

_____

_____

# Medical T (TIPs) #8 - Penis Pilates

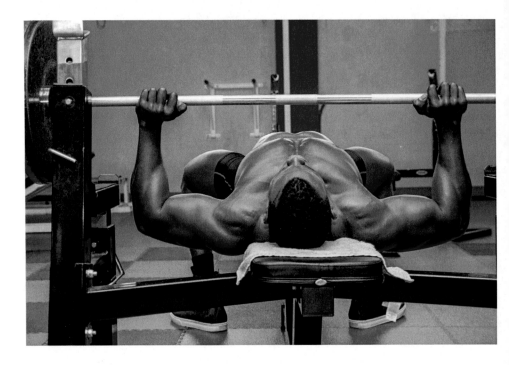

#GYNEGirls, go get your man right now because y'all both need to read this chapter together. We're going to have a chat about ways to make his penis work better.

First of all, men need to have regular erections. SO GET TO WACKING OFF #GENTS! If you don't, your manhood could shrink by 1-2 centimeters.

Know what else can help? Exercising helps work out the penis too; it will boost your testosterone. Hitting up the gym will also make you feel better NAKED. Ladies, you know men are all about confidence. Sorry fellas, but it's the truth. While in the gym work on those core muscles. These muscles are connected to your penis muscles. Have any of you ever met a man that can make his penis jump when it's hard? Dr. Drai has... Hello! That means he has a strong core...AND a strong penis. LOL! Here's my Favorite "Medical T": Don't forget about your Kegels!

That's right you heard what I said. Kegels aren't just for women. #GENTS, here's how you do it. When you start to pee, stop the stream for 10 seconds and then let it flow. You can do this every time you whip it out! This will help to get your penis nice and strong. Go, #GENTs, Go!

#GYNEGirls additionally, get rid of the alcohol—that's a no brainer. He needs to stop smoking as well. Puffing makes his penis get smaller. Tell your BOO he has to lose weight too. Fluffier men have lower levels of testosterone. In addition to eliminating alcohol he also needs to learn to lower his stress level. His cock won't work right if he is too focused on other things. Also, make sure he gets plenty of sleep and is eating healthy. Low cholesterol and low sugar diets are best. However, he CAN eat dark chocolate; it helps keep his _ICK hard. But enough with the penis pilates!

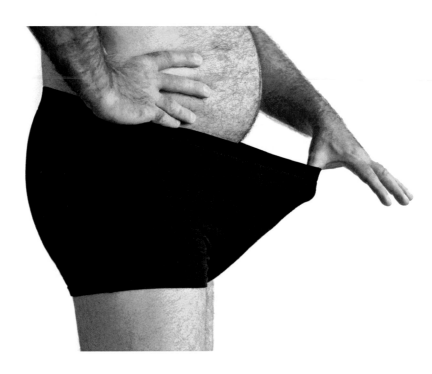

# MEDICAL T NOTES

_____

_____

_____

_____

_____

_____

_____

_____

_____

_____

_____

_____

# MEDICAL ☕ NOTES

_____

_____

_____

_____

_____

_____

_____

_____

_____

_____

_____

_____

_____

_____

# Medical T (TIPs) #9 - Condom Sense Isn't Too Common

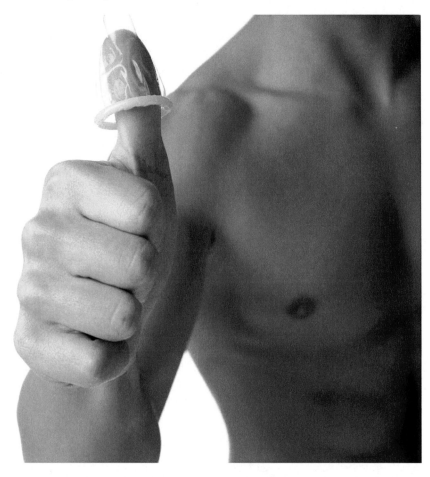

I need to teach you #GYNEGirls how to pick a condom for your #GENT. You prolly have NEVER heard this #DrDraiMedicalT before. Your #GENT is clueless too. If I teach YOU, you can teach HIM. Get it, got it, GOOD!

First of all, Dr. Drai LOVES the male condom. If the condom FITS, YOU will not get #Preggo or catch a #STI BECAUSE it won't slip off or break. Condoms are sized in length and girth (width or thickness). The girth is more important than the length.

Let's go over some tricks for you to pick the right condom to properly FIT your man's penis. Measure the girth (thickness) of his penis when it's erect.

If his girth is less than 4.7 inches wide, he needs a snug fit condom. Try Beyond Seven Studded or Glyde Slim Fit. If his girth is between 4.7 to 5.1 inches wide, he can use a regular fit condom. Try Lifestyles Skyn or Durex PleasureMax. If his girth is between 5.1 to 6 inches wide, chile he needs a larger fit condom. #SizeQueens, can I get an AMEN! Try Trojan Magnums or the FC2 condom (the female condom). Just take the inner thick ring out of the female condom and it turns into a male condom. Cool right? Now that is some juicy Medical T don't you agree!

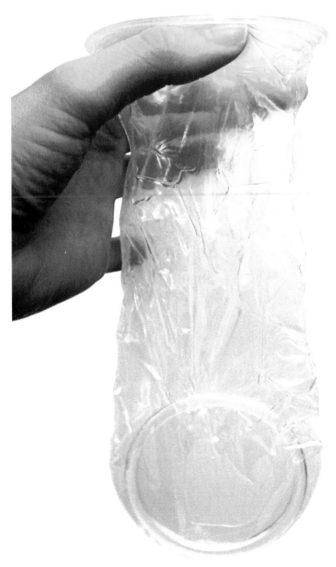

In case you don't have a measuring tape handy, don't worry. You can also check his penile GIRTH by putting his erect penis in an empty toilet paper roll. To measure, use these simple guidelines: If there's too much room in the roll, he's a snugger fit. If his penis fits comfortably in the roll, he's a regular fit. If his penis can't fit in the roll, he's large. That's pretty simple right?

Be careful #GYNEGirls. Please have some condom sense... Always have three different size condoms with you at all times. You never know if your new guy will have a small, medium, or large penis. Another reason I want you to learn how to pick the right size condom for your #GENT is because I DON'T TRUST THEM. You should practice putting a condom on a banana before you get TOO EXCITED when you see the REAL THANG. Practice makes PERFECT.

Here's my FAVORITE "Medical T. Use only water-based or silicone lube with latex condoms, i.e. OIL will cause damage. No Vaseline fellas!

# MEDICAL ☕ NOTES

_____

_____

_____

_____

_____

_____

_____

_____

_____

_____

_____

_____

_____

# MEDICAL NOTES

_____

_____

_____

_____

_____

_____

_____

_____

_____

_____

_____

_____

_____

# Medical T (TIPs) #10 - The Benefits of Jackin' Off

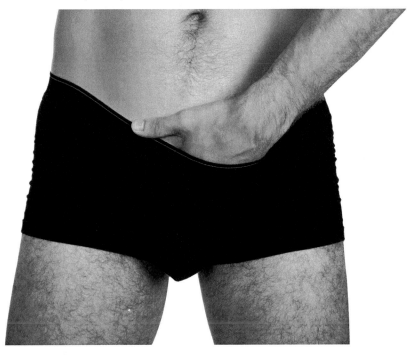

Seven out of ten adult men masturbate. Most #GENTs learn how to jerk their chicken fast and in silence; teens are always worried about their mom walking in on them. So embarrassing!

Although, masturbation can be seen as a cause for shame for some, it has some great benefits. Here's my FAVORITE "Medical T." One of the biggest benefits of jackin' off is that it reduces your risk of prostate cancer in men over age 50 as long as they ejaculate (nut) at least 1 to 2 times a week. On the flip side, men in their 20s and 30s who masturbated 2 to 7 times per week have a higher risk of developing prostate cancer.

Let's crack the NUT open and talk about orgasms. #GENTs, when you BURST, you will have uncontrolled muscle contractions in your penis and anus. Then your body releases dopamine, which makes you feel happy. Your heart rate increases, you breathe heavier, your blood pressure increases, and your entire body gets flushed due to norepinephrine.

Serotonin is then released making you sleepy. Ladies, now you know why your #GENT falls right to sleep after he ejaculates. Having an orgasm makes him both happy and helps him get some good sleep! The body is SO amazing right? #GENTs if you're not making your girl fall asleep, she may be faking the Big O.

Masturbation has many other great benefits. It helps your penis get and stay hard, relieves stress, beats depression, boosts your immune system, makes you smarter, helps you live longer, makes you look younger, AND helps fight heart disease!

Masturbation also gives you a chance to examine your penis, balls, and anus to check for signs of STI's and signs of cancer as mentioned in the introduction. And fellas, guess what? You can't get your girl #Preggo or catch a STI! And NO, you won't go BLIND, LOL!

Use lube when you jack off to prevent chapped skin. See, there are benefits of masturbation.

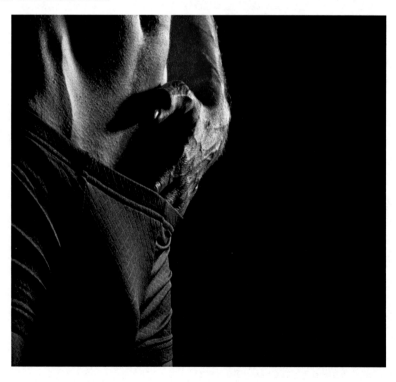

# MEDICAL NOTES

_____

_____

_____

_____

_____

_____

_____

_____

_____

_____

_____

_____

_____

# MEDICAL ☕ NOTES

_____

_____

_____

_____

_____

_____

_____

_____

_____

_____

_____

_____

_____

# Medical T (TIPs) #11 - The Ultimate Hard-On

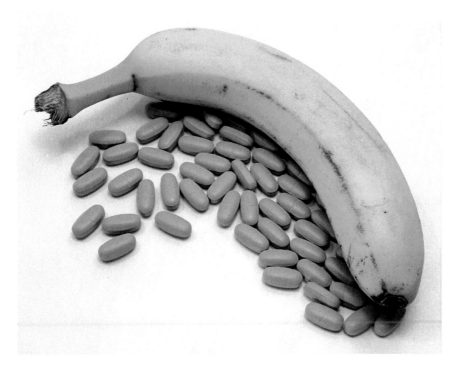

#GENTs, for some of you this situation is all too real: You are in your 30s and you finally meet that one woman you want to settle down with. You have been dating her for three months now and it's finally time to knock her boots off in the bedroom so YOU can close the deal. Dr. Drai gets it!

To make sure you bring your "A Game", you decide to "BORROW" some Cialis (tadalafil) or Viagra (sildenafil) from your uncle or dad, OR worse, purchase these pills over the Internet. You take them and you DO knock her socks off. After you both orgasm, she wants to cuddle. A couple of hours have passed and your penis starts to hurt; and I mean BAD. She notices that your piece isn't soft yet. She freaks out and wants you to go to the ER immediately. Long story short...you finally have to admit to the ER DOC (and your girl) that you took Viagra (sildenafil). This story happens OOOH too often.

PLEASE don't take meds that your doctor didn't prescribe for you. Taking medications like Viagra (sildenafil), Cialis (tadalafil), and Levitra (vardenafil) can have side effects and result in what's known as Priapism.

Priapism is a persistent erection for more than 4 hours. After you nut, blood should drain from the penis making it soft. In this condition, the blood is trapped for some reason. If you don't seek help, your penis may not work anymore. Sickle cell anemia, leukemia, medications like Wellbutrin (bupropion), Prozac (fluoxetine), and Coumadin (warfarin sodium) OR smoking "Mary Jane" can also cause this.

In order to make the erection go away, your DOC will put ice packs on your penis, numb it and aspirate the blood with a needle, or you may have to go to surgery. Is all of this worth it to impress a girl? No. Here's my Favorite "Medical T": To make him last longer, try the start-stop technique #GYNEGirls. Start having sex with your #BAE. Take a break i.e. have him pull out before he climaxes. Then repeat.

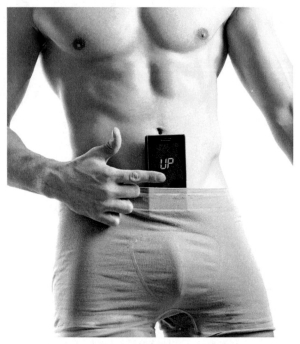

*BTW #Gents stop putting your laptop on your junk, this can affect your testosterone production.*

# MEDICAL ☕ NOTES

_____

_____

_____

_____

_____

_____

_____

_____

_____

_____

_____

_____

_____

_____

# MEDICAL NOTES

_____

_____

_____

_____

_____

_____

_____

_____

_____

_____

_____

_____

_____

## Medical T (TIPs) #12 - Blue Ball Blues

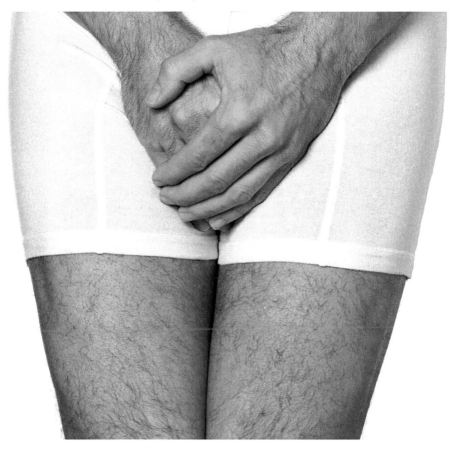

You ladies ask me this question at least once a week. Are "blue balls" a real thing? Your man really has convinced you that you can give him blue balls. STOP believing the hype! "Blue balls" happen when your man has an erection for a long time but doesn't ejaculate. It's not harmful. AND his balls DO NOT turn blue.

During an erection, there's an increase of blood flow in the penis, which causes pressure. If the pressure is not released, his nuts can hurt. Chile it is not that serious. He can give himself a helping hand (WINK!) OR just wait it out. You know #GENTs can be babies sometimes. Here's my Favorite "Medical T": The next time he complains tell him Dr. Drai said to start playing with himself. He'll be quiet; you know THEY can't live without the vagina. The straight ones of course...

Since we are on the subject of balls, let me clear up a couple of other things. The right testicle is LARGER than the left. The left testicle hangs LOWER than the other. Ya'll ask me that all the time too. I'm so over blue balls. Let's move on. NEXT!

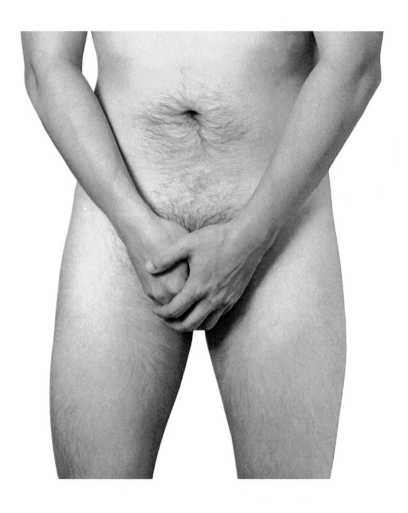

# MEDICAL ☕ NOTES

_____

_____

_____

_____

_____

_____

_____

_____

_____

_____

_____

_____

_____

# MEDICAL ☕ NOTES

_____

_____

_____

_____

_____

_____

_____

_____

_____

_____

_____

_____

_____

## Medical T (TIPs) #13 - Morning Wood Mishaps

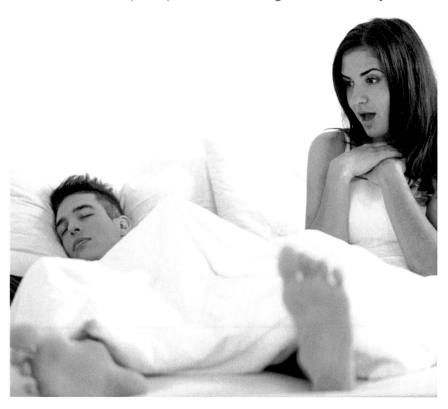

#GYNEGirls, we have all seen it. Most of you use it to see how BIG your man's thang is. It's called nocturnal penile tumescence, aka morning wood. Here's how this works.

During the REM phase of sleep (which is the DEEP sleep), your #GENT's penis gets hard. There are two hormones that are working here: Norepinephrine (NE) and Testosterone (T). NE actually causes the penis vessels to vasoconstrict, which means not fill with blood (penis is soft). T causes the penis vessels to vasodialate meaning fill with blood (penis is hard). That's why men with lots of testosterone are always HORNY!!!

Have you ever been spooning with your man and all of a sudden you feel a LOG on your back? We have all been there, #GYNEGirls. During the DREAM sleep, NE lowers and T increases; the penis fills with blood and an erection occurs. Your #BAE may have 3-4 erections while sleeping per night AND that's completely normal.

In addition, the bladder also fills with urine while he is sleeping which can cause the penis to become hard as well. Here's my Favorite "Medical T": If your man doesn't have morning wood, he may have an issue down there. You should encourage him to talk to a DOC about this. NEXT chapter!

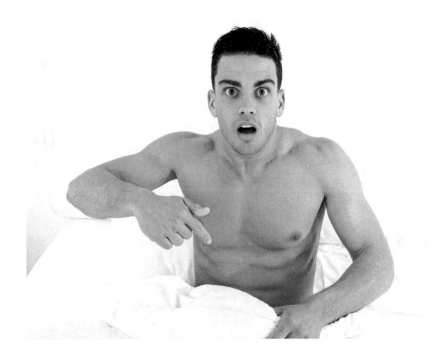

# MEDICAL NOTES

_____

_____

_____

_____

_____

_____

_____

_____

_____

_____

_____

_____

_____

# MEDICAL NOTES

_____

_____

_____

_____

_____

_____

_____

_____

_____

_____

_____

_____

_____

_____

## Medical T (TIPs) #14 - Big Balls Galore

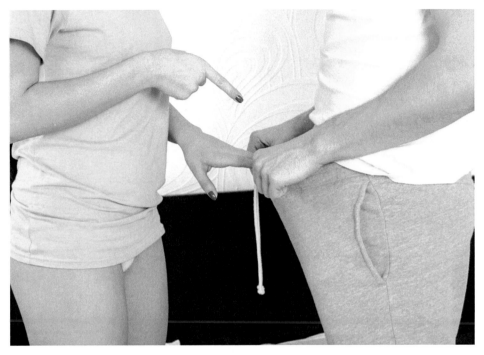

#GYNEGirls, y'all love to talk about how size matters when it comes to the penis, but you are missing out on sizing up the balls. LOL!

Have you ever seen testicles that were as big as coconuts? Neither have I. The average testicle is about 2 to 3 inches in length and 1 inch in width. I told you this before. The right is usually LARGER than the left, but the left one hangs lower. Let me get back on subject.

Several scientific papers have been published about this BIG phenomenon and here's what we know thus far. Women are more likely to cheat on a guy if he has big testicles. Men with big balls have a higher chance for heart disease, especially if they already have sexual dysfunction. Here's my Favorite "Medical T": men with smaller balls make better dads. Yeah! That's a plus. See ladies, size does matter. Just maybe not in the way you thought.

# MEDICAL NOTES

_____

_____

_____

_____

_____

_____

_____

_____

_____

_____

_____

_____

_____

# MEDICAL NOTES

_____

_____

_____

_____

_____

_____

_____

_____

_____

_____

_____

_____

_____

## Medical T (TIPs) #15 -My Anaconda Don't...

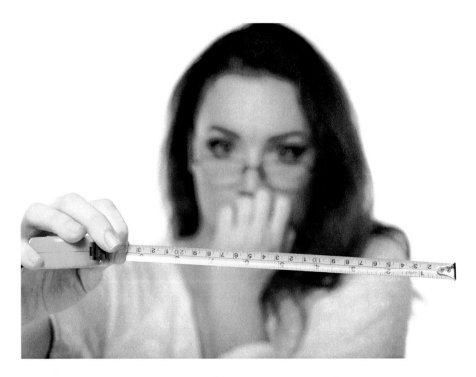

The largest (recorded) penis is 9.5 inches soft and 13.5 inches hard. Oh and he's not a black man. Chile I'm sweatin' just thinking about that. #GYNEGirls, I know some of the SIZE QUEENs out there love the friction of a big penis, but you need to be careful! Sometimes a larger penis may tear the vagina and cause bleeding. Not good! And then you have to have emergency surgery to fix your lady parts! So embarrassing...a large penis can cause sex to be painful. Also NOT GOOD! That defeats your purpose of having sex in the first place, right?

Here's my FAVORITE "Medical T": If you have a Mr. BIG, ride him so you can control how much is going in your lady part. That missionary position can be a BEAST with an ANACONDA chile.

The vagina CAN stretch, but try not to take advantage of that MEDICAL "T" TIP! You need to use water-based lubricants (Astroglide is my favorite) especially when the penis, dildo, or vibrator is larger than your vagina. And, yes, I said dildo and vibrator! You can also use a vibrator on the underside of his penis when giving him head. You already know you can't BOB that whole thang.

Hunni we got to be creative with those long ones. LOL!

Stop blushing! Oh and BTW studies say the ladies who date men with BIG penises cheat. To my Mr. BIGs out there, it doesn't matter how BIG you are DOWN THERE if you are not warming up her mind. Remember, fellas, sex is cerebral with women. Step your FOREPLAY game up.

FOREPLAY doesn't just start in the bedroom. Here are some suggestions: weekly date nights, surprise lunch dates, send her flowers at work, get the kids ready for school, and cook dinner sometimes. You get the picture, fellas. The more you turn her on, the more her vagina will get wet. And that big thang you are rockin' will SLIDE right in. SPLASH...LOL!

One more thing, ladies, stop looking at his crotch to determine the size of his penis. LOOK AT HIS FINGERS, girl! There was a small study that revealed the greater the difference in length between a man's ring finger when compared to his index finger, the longer the length of his penis. Hunni in my experience, TALL, SKINNY men always have the ANACONDAs. But remember ladies, sometimes the best lovers don't wear golds.

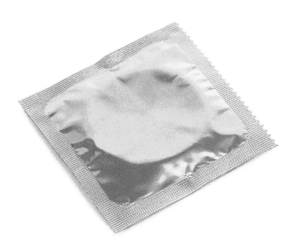

# MEDICAL NOTES

_____

_____

_____

_____

_____

_____

_____

_____

_____

_____

_____

_____

_____

_____

# MEDICAL NOTES

_____

_____

_____

_____

_____

_____

_____

_____

_____

_____

_____

_____

# Medical T (TIPs) #16 -Growers And Show(ers)

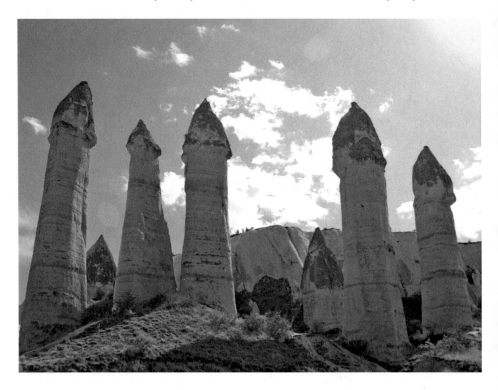

Penises come in all shapes AND sizes. But, #GYNEGIrls—you already know this #DrDraiMedicalT...at least I hope so. There are banana shaped ones (curved up), ones with mushroom heads, the Number 2 (aka Mr. Pencil), the Chode (short/fatty), Mr. Ripped (the ones with the BIG veins), the HOOK (curved down) and of course the Anaconda and Mr. Small. There are too, Too, TOO MANY to count!

I haven't seen a twin yet. Speaking of twins, there is such a thing as having 2 penises. It's called Diphallia or Penile Duplication (PD). 1 in 5 million men have this condition but, let's not get side tracked here... back to the subject at hand AND my FAVORITE "Medical T."

Now, Mr. Small is always going to be good at oral sex. He's perfected the art of pleasing you without using his penis. The banana-shaped ones are great for missionary style sex. The curve helps make him touch YOUR G-spot. But let me get back on subject ONCE AGAIN- there are really only 2 types of penises though.

The Growers and the Show(ers). Growers are penises that expand and lengthen when it gets hard. Show(ers) are penises that are already big; when they get hard they don't get much bigger. Do you prefer a Grower or a Show(er) ladies? #TeamShow(er) over here. Let me know what you werkin' with from the jump. LOL!

Most #GENTs are GROWers – over 70% of them. Once again, there are no studies that correlate how much a man's penis will grow once aroused. So stop stressing GUYS! When she finally sees your penis, it will be erect anyway.

Next chapter!

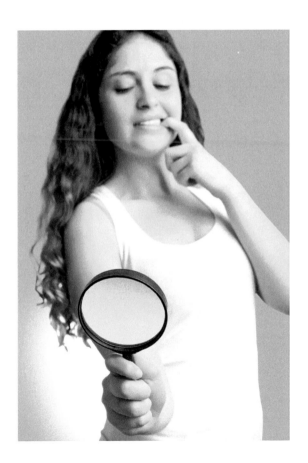

# MEDICAL NOTES

_____

_____

_____

_____

_____

_____

_____

_____

_____

_____

_____

_____

_____

_____

# MEDICAL ☕ NOTES

_____

_____

_____

_____

_____

_____

_____

_____

_____

_____

_____

_____

_____

## Medical T (TIPs) #17 -To Spit or to Swallow

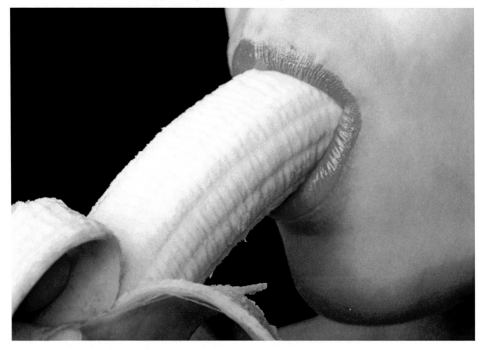

Now let's get REAL. You ladies are always asking me if you should swallow his nut. These #Gents out here are convincing ya'll that swallowing is an act of LOVE. They even have you #GYNEGirls thinking that their semen tastes good. Don't fall for this chile. Let's talk about ejaculate first... you know – CUM. For some reason, you seem obsessed with it too. SMH...

I'm glad that we have already learned in the INTRO that sperm and semen are not the same. Just to let you know, ladies, the usual ejaculate is about ½ of a teaspoon. There's about 200 million sperm in that ½ of a teaspoon too. WOW!

BTW there's only about 5-25 calories in it depending on the amount he cums. The cool thing about sperm is that it only takes 2 months for your #BAE to make NEW ones.

Be careful-#GENTs can make sperm forever. Have you ever seen a 30+ year old female pregnant with her 70+ year old man's baby? I have...too many times. Plus sperm can live in the vagina for up to 6 days. So if you are going to have unprotected sex with multiple men please space them out. I know you have heard about TWINS born with 2 different dads? SIDE EYE I know that's not you because you know to always use condoms RIGHT?

Here's my FAVORITE "Medical T." Lots of you #GENTs ask how can you make a lot more semen. The answer is pace out your orgasms, let your store build up. To make good sperm (you know, if you ACTUALLY want to have a baby), you should also keep your nuts cool and hanging. Limit wearing briefs, crossing your legs, and getting in hot tubs. These situations can all affect your soldiers.

Now let's get down to this Medical T. There are no studies that tell us how to make his semen taste better. It's been postulated that if he eats asparagus, red meat or dairy, his semen will taste bad. I have also HEARD from patients that if he eats lots of sweet fruits like pineapples and kiwi his semen will taste sweeter. It's all hearsay ladies... It does make sense though. So to answer the question, to spit or to swallow? NEITHER! Can you say STIs? Since you are using condoms when having oral sex there should be nothing to swallow right? Ladies a TRUE act of LOVE is when a #Gent puts on a condom because he wants to protect you. Don't forget that. Next chapter!

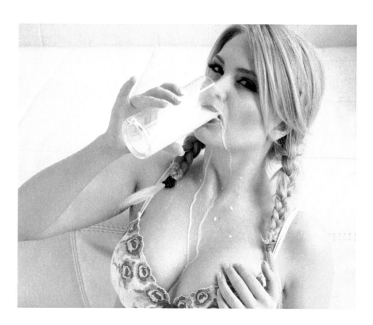

# MEDICAL NOTES

_____

_____

_____

_____

_____

_____

_____

_____

_____

_____

_____

_____

# MEDICAL NOTES

_____

_____

_____

_____

_____

_____

_____

_____

_____

_____

_____

_____

_____

# Medical T (TIPs) #18 -Limp _ick

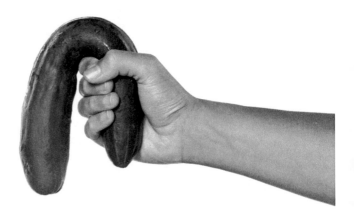

Erectile dysfunction (ED) or impotence means a man is unable to get an erection or keep an erection during sex. 18 million men suffer from this condition, ladies. There are lots of causes—medications, chronic illnesses, poor blood flow to the penis, drinking too much alcohol, testosterone too low or even being too tired.

Let's discuss some natural ways to cope with a man who can't get it up or keep it up. First of all, don't make him feel like he's less than a man, ladies. You know how y'all can get. And stop discussing and comparing your sex lives with your girlfriends. Try to keep this just between you two.

Try to spice things up a little, Have more FOREPLAY. Try Oral Sex. ORAL just doesn't mean the penis ladies. Play with his nipples or the back of his neck. KISS him more. Add sex toys in the bedroom BUT make sure they are smaller than his penis. I keep repeating this one because ya'll keep ignoring me.

You should also get his diabetes, cholesterol, and/or high blood pressure under control. Make him quit smoking, and make sure he doesn't drink alcohol. He should do MORE cardio exercises and find ways to reduce his stress and anxiety levels. Be sure he is getting enough sleep and eating a balanced diet; cook for him ladies.

There are nitrates in leafy greens and beets, flavonoids in dark chocolate,

protein in pistachios, and antioxidants in watermelon. Chile, Beyonce KNEW
the secret. There are lycopene in tomatoes and grapefruit AND zinc in oysters.
All of these important nutrients will help his limp _ick.

Taking supplements like ginseng or ginkgo may also help. Has your
man ever gone to the corner store and bought back those "Sex Pills"? They have
ginseng and ginkgo in them. Interesting, right? DON'T let him take those pills
though, ladies. You never know what else is in them. Get the trusted ones from a
local pharmacy, And BE patient! You two will work this out.

Here's my FAVORITE "Medical T": In addition to all of these try my

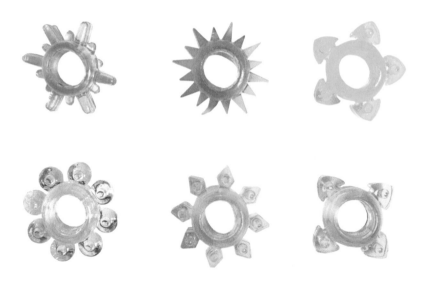

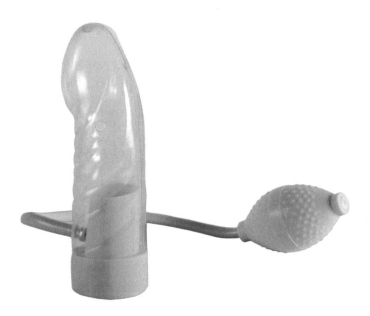

fave solution; Have him wear a cock ring. Have you ever been to a male strip club? I know you have. The strippers get their penises semi-hard backstage (fluffed) and then they put cock rings around their balls and penis to make their manhood stay semi-hard throughout their performance. This can work for your BOO, too. You can buy cock rings at an adult store or order them online. They usually come three in one pack.

Oh! You can also try a vacuum penis pump to help him maintain his thickness. Do the natural thing first BEFORE you try medications like Cialis (tadalafil), Viagra (sildenafil), or Levitra (Vardenafil HCl). You want to avoid any possible side effects.

# MEDICAL NOTES

_____

_____

_____

_____

_____

_____

_____

_____

_____

_____

_____

_____

_____

_____

# MEDICAL NOTES

_____

_____

_____

_____

_____

_____

_____

_____

_____

_____

_____

_____

_____

## Medical T (TIPs) #19 - The Short Short Man

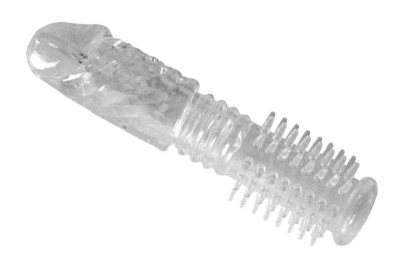

Sing it with me: "Eeny, weeny, teeny, weeny, shriveled little short short man. Don't want, Don't want, Don't want. Don't want no short short man." #GYNEGirls, you know you AND your girlfriends have dated and have had sympathy sex with a man with a small one. You #SizeQueens that are reading this out there are clutching your pearls right now. LOL! I get it, THE HORROR right?

A micro-penis (aka the short, short man) is less than 1.6 inches soft and 3 inches hard. Traction devices can be used or surgery can be done to make his penis longer. BTW, penises do shrink as you age. #GENTs, Dr. Drai knows how to get you in the gym. If you lose weight, your cock will LOOK bigger.

For you good-hearted orators don't neglect your little man. Give him some head! That way he won't be self-conscious. He will definitely love you. Throw that lube in the trash (or stash it for your next BIG boo LOL!). Hunni he will be sliding everywhere but the right place. Here's my FAVORITE "Medical T": The best positions for you to get yours if dating a short short man are modified missionary with your pelvis tilted up in the air and your legs crisscrossed. This position will give your man maximum access and it also makes your vagina smaller. Win-Win situation.

Fellas if this is you, buy a penis extender. A penis extender is a device that makes your meat longer and has ridges along it that will make your woman feel good. You can buy one from a sex store or online. But, a word of caution, PLEASE learn to use it before trying it out on your woman. Last BUT not least, if you are not as well endowed, try ANAL; that hole is USUALLY MUCH smaller. Don't forget the lube. Next chapter!

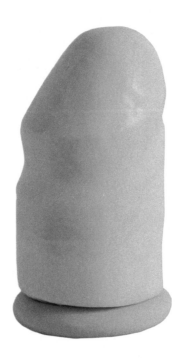

# MEDICAL NOTES

_____

_____

_____

_____

_____

_____

_____

_____

_____

_____

_____

_____

_____

# MEDICAL ☕ NOTES

_____

_____

_____

_____

_____

_____

_____

_____

_____

_____

_____

_____

_____

_____

# Medical T (TIPs) #20 -Pre-Cum Penalties

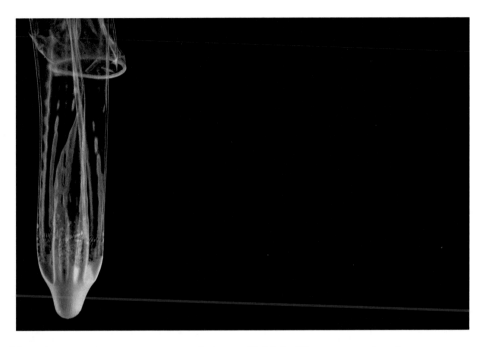

Now this issue is more common than we all think. If your man ejaculates sooner during sexual intercourse than he expects and he is frustrated about it, he suffers from premature ejaculation (PE) aka pre-cum. He's so upset about this that he avoids all sexual activity. Most of the time these fellas can't delay cumming for more than 1 minute after entry into your lady part.

We don't really know what causes PE; it could be relationship problems, stress, anxiety, or even thyroid problems. Counseling is a must, ladies. You can't make him go. He will see a therapist when he's ready.

Here are some sexual techniques to help him out. Have him masturbate and train himself not to nut. He can do this by Squeezing the area between the head AND shaft of his penis until the sensation passes. Then have him go back to masturbating. The same technique can be done when ya'll are knocking the boots too. Oh, and don't forget Kegels! Like I said, they are not just for women.

This will help strengthen his pelvic muscles. Medications such as Paxil (paroxetine), Zoloft (sertraline), Prozac (fluoxetine) or numbing cream that you put on his penis can also be used as a treatment. The new medication on the market for PE is Promescent; it's a topical spray applied to the penis 10 minutes before having sex.

Let me get back on track here... Pre-cum has been medically examined and we found out that the fluid has dead or no sperm at all. However, it is possible for small amounts of LIVE sperm to find their way into pre-ejaculate. Here's my FAVORITE "Medical T." Sperm can be left behind from a previous ejaculation, meaning LIVE ones can be released into pre-cum. That's why #GENTs should urinate between ejaculations to wash out the leftover sperm. The withdrawal method can fail because of leftover sperm in pre-cum. So strap it up! It's better to be safe than sorry RIGHT?
#Condoms

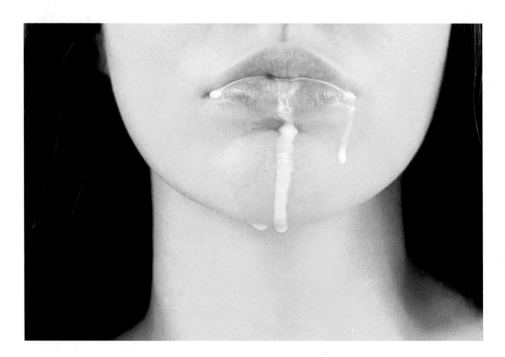

# MEDICAL ☕ NOTES

_____

_____

_____

_____

_____

_____

_____

_____

_____

_____

_____

_____

_____

_____

# MEDICAL ☕ NOTES

_____

_____

_____

_____

_____

_____

_____

_____

_____

_____

_____

# Bonus: Tips for Oral Sex

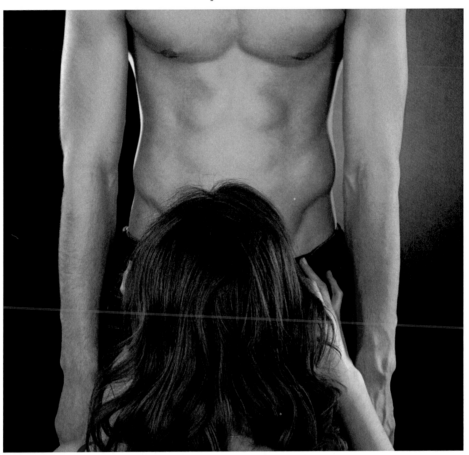

#GYNEGirls, are you ready for this Medical T? Let's get some basic terms out of the way. Cunnilingus is a fancy word for sex performed orally on "lady parts" and fellatio is another fancy word for oral sex performed on "man parts."

To be good at oral sex #GYNEGirls, you need to observe the art and practice the art. Watch porn. Yes PORN isn't just for men ladies. Practice on a dildo or your MM (maintenance man). LOL! Stay hydrated; drink plenty of water. This helps you make enough saliva. No man wants dry head. Slurp away- they love the noise. My oral sex tips are below. They are not in any kind of order. Enjoy!

# 20 Bonus Oral Sex Tips

1. Go easy with the teeth! Ouch!

2. You definitely should try to deep throat. But BEWARE: That gag reflex is REAL. So practice, practice, practice... practice makes perfect. WINK! To start, place the tip of your tongue on the roof of your mouth. Then let his penis hit the underside of your tongue. This makes him THINK you are DEEP THROATING.

3. Use your tongue to swirl around the penis especially the head.

4. Like I told you before...Don't ignore his other manly parts- the underside of the penis is very sensitive – lick it! The area between his anus and testes is sensitive– the MALE G-spot. Men have nipples too ladies. Massage his testes while going to town on the penis shaft.

5. If he's uncut, tease the foreskin gently! Tickle the inside of his foreskin with your tongue.

6. Be spontaneous! Whip it out in the car, at the park, at the beach. GO IN! Try sucking him off in the dark. Better yet, when he walks in the door from work, drop to your knees AND get to WERK.

7. Try rimming his rectum. Make sure he showers before. Men aren't as clean as you ladies! You don't want any surprises.

8. Suck him off in the mirror so he can see you at all angles! Men are so vain!

9. Definitely let him touch you when you are giving him head; let him play with your nipples, G-spot or CLIT. That's HOT!

10. Put something cold in your mouth like ice cubes right before you go down; he'll love it. Try mint or champagne also, they have the same affect.

*Oral Sex FUN Fact: 1 out of 400 men are flexible enough to give himself oral pleasure. Now that is Interesting!*

11. If you are tired of sucking, give him a hand job with some lube. Or let him smack his penis on your face.

12. Play with his urethral meatus (pee hole). Stick your tongue in there and apply some pressure.

13. Make good eye contact.

14. Lick that line in the middle of his nut sack; it's called the raphe. That's a hot spot.

15. Put his balls in your mouth one by one and suck lightly. Stroke his shaft at the same time.

16. If he will let you, play with his prostate. Finger him- use lube.

17. Use your tongue to play with the ridge of the penis- the place where the head meets the shaft.

18. Talk dirty to him. Tell him what you want him to do to your body.

19. Do this trick. Right before he nuts, grab his balls and tug down gently. This heightens his orgasm.

20. My favorite tip ladies is for you to grab the penis, put one hand on top of the other and gently twist in opposite directions AND up and down. Suck the tip at the same dang time. YASSS! Make sure you lube up the shaft.

You gotta use condoms #GYNEGirls! Spice it up and use flavored ones! Lots of the girls rave about chocolate. DO NOT put a flavored condom in your vagina or rectum! It's just for ORAL play! Use dental dam for rimming and latex gloves for fingering.

# MEDICAL NOTES

_____

_____

_____

_____

_____

_____

_____

_____

_____

_____

_____

_____

_____

# MEDICAL ☕ NOTES

_____

_____

_____

_____

_____

_____

_____

_____

_____

_____

_____

_____

_____

_____

# Thank You

Thank you #GYNEGirls, #Preggos, and #GENTs from the bottom of my heart for purchasing and reading this book. This is my second one - would love your feedback. Don't be scared; I can take it. I hope you have learned some NEW things about the penis. It's an amazing organ, isn't it? Thanks again for supporting my fight against domestic violence. 1 in 4 women will experience domestic violence in her lifetime. Unfortunately, most domestic violence incidents are never reported. Your book purchase will help make a difference. Spread the word!

You know Dr. Drai is super busy! I'm either seeing a patient in one of the 8 offices I work in, in surgery in 1 of the 2 hospitals I operate in, catching a baby, doing an online, print, radio, or TV media interview or on the lecture circuit educating DOCs about new trends in women's health. You are tired just reading this...I have some exciting news for you ladies. Soon Dr. Drai will exclusively be traveling the country taking care of women that need focused attention. He may be in a city near you. Let's stay connected so I can keep you updated on my activities. Here's how- click on the links below:

Website: http://DrDrai.com
Facebook: https://www.facebook.com/DrDraiOBGYN
Twitter: https://twitter.com/DrDraiOBGYN
You Tube: http://www.youtube.com/user/DrDraiOBGYN
Instagram: http://instagram.com/DrDraiOBGYN
Pinterest: http://www.pinterest.com/DrDraiOBGYN
LinkedIn: https://www.linkedin.com/in/DrDraiOBGYN
Google+: https://www.google.com/+DrDraiOBGYN

# About Dr. Drai

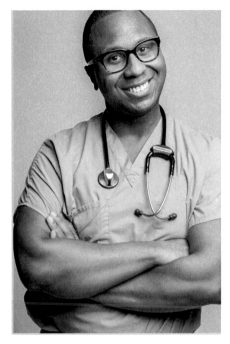

Dr. Draion M. Burch, DO (Dr. Drai) a highly respected, board-certified Obstetrician and Gynecologist, is a nationally-recognized author, speaker, consultant, and go-to media expert on women's health and transgender health issues.

He travels the country to meet with women one-on-one and in groups to provide and instruct on healthcare. Although Dr. Drai may be requested to spread his medical expertise to all four corners of the U.S., he always makes time to genuinely help those in need.
Dr. Drai is a pragmatic physician who offers endless charisma, high energy, and a larger-than-life personality. His "bedside manner" makes it obvious why his patients have named him "America's OBGYN."

Dr. Drai is the founder and chief medical advisor of DrDrai.com, where he discusses actionable ideas and real-world strategies to help women take control of their health. As an openly gay gynecologist he has patients flocking to him and his website for not only his medical expertise, but because of the security they feel in the way he cares for, relates to, and teaches them. His upbeat personality and genuine concern helps women feel at ease coming to him about subjects ranging from embarrassing vaginal care to serious sexual assault.

His mission: Real medical advice, simplified.

Dr. Drai takes his unique brand to the camera on his YouTube channel to spill his popular "Medical T" (TIPS) helping his self-titled #Preggos, #GYNEGirls and #GENTs pursue a healthier life. Dr. Drai's on-point advice on off-the-wall questions about sexual health issues has many calling him a "sexpert." Dr. Drai earned his Bachelor of Science degree from Xavier University of Louisiana, Doctorate of Osteopathic Medicine degree from The Ohio University and completed his internship and residency at Michigan State University.

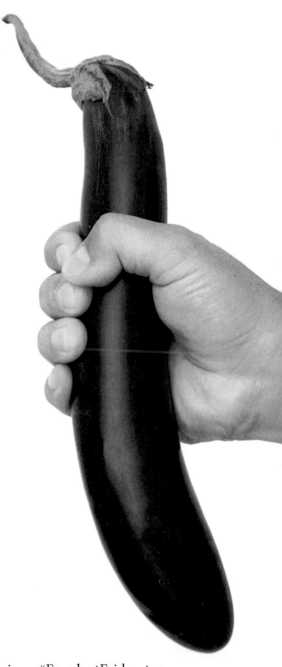

#GYNEGirls & #GENTs, Dr. Drai misses #EggplantFriday, too.

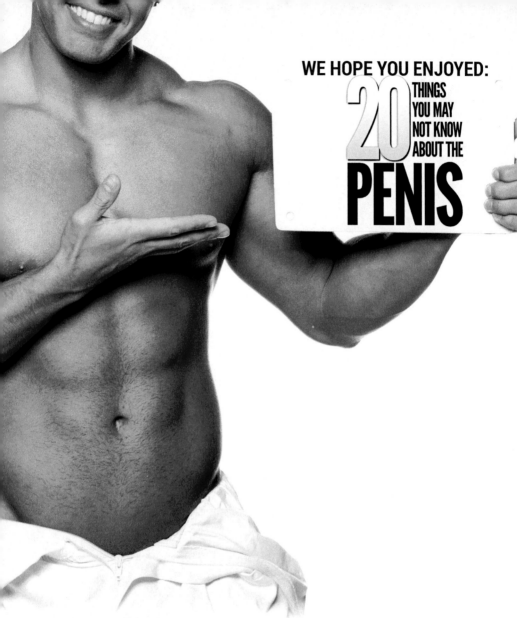

WE HOPE YOU ENJOYED:

# 20 THINGS YOU MAY NOT KNOW ABOUT THE

# PENIS

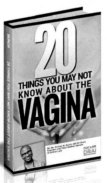

Because you have contributed to a cause dear to Dr. Drai's heart, he has created a free book for you as a Thank You.

To download, "20 Things You May Not Know About the Vagina," today visit:

## DrDrai.com/Vagina

Made in the USA
Middletown, DE
22 November 2015